Pokes, Pinches, and Loose Wires

By Lizzie Bell

Illustrated by: Ray Jean Cottle

Face of a Champion® Multi-Media Literacy Program
Copyright© 2012 Kbella and Company, LLC

ISBN: 978-0-9801855-9-1

Used with Permission of: John P. Bell Family Foundation
All rights reserved, including the right of reproduction in whole or in part in any form.

When it comes to books… think Out of the Box!

Out of the Box Books
P.O. Box 64878
Tucson, AZ 85728
www.outoftheboxbooks.com

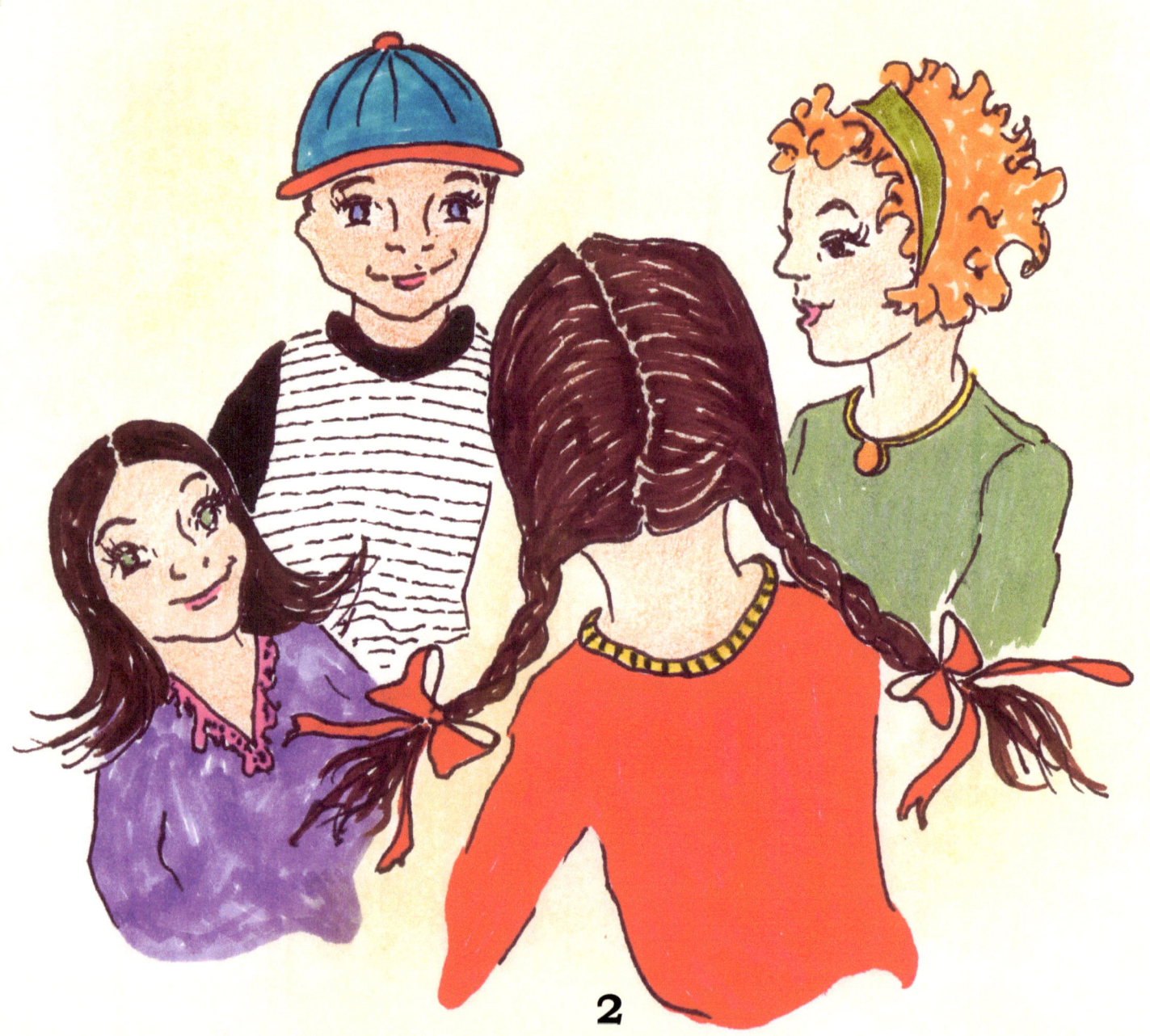

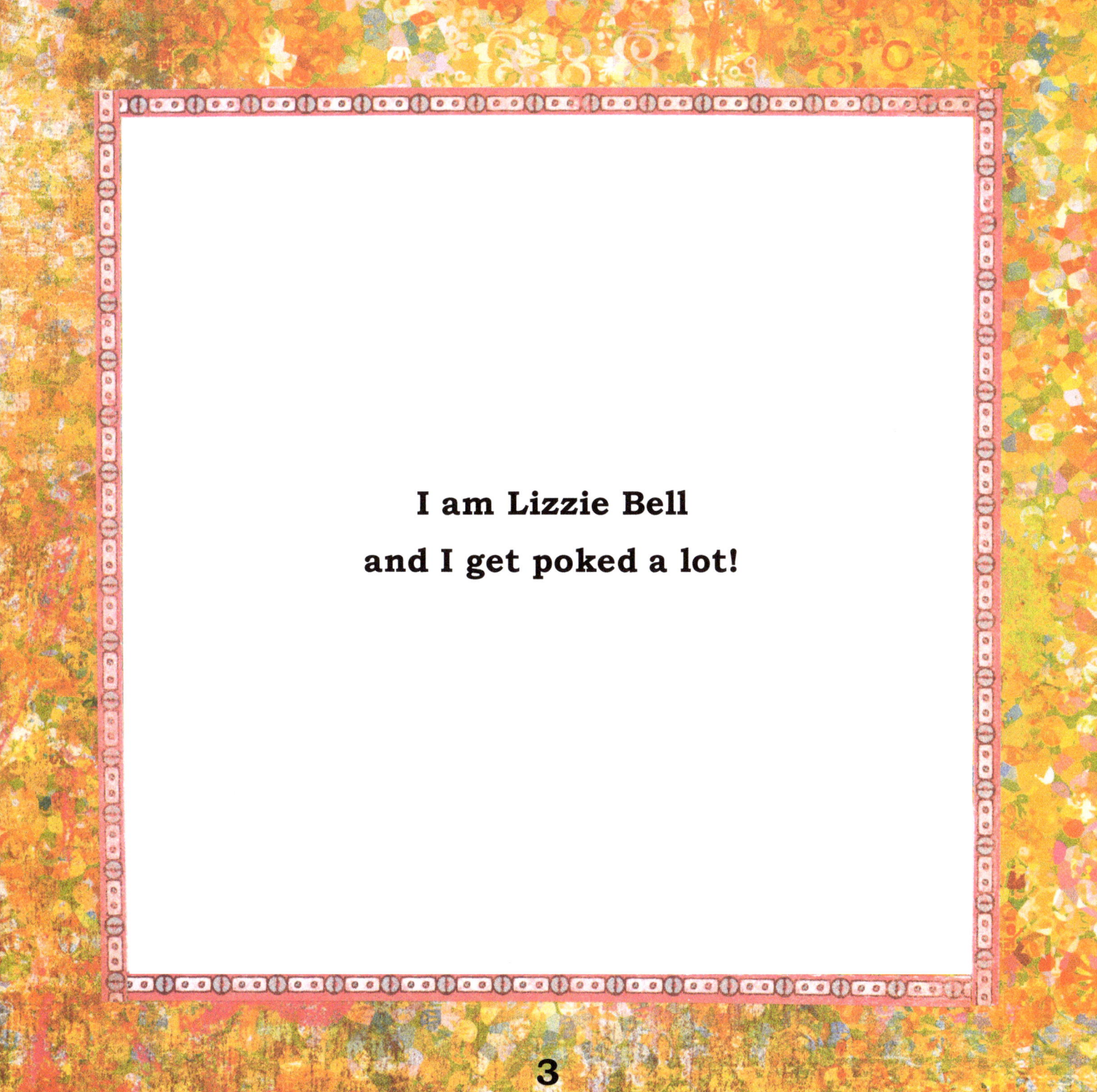

I am Lizzie Bell
and I get poked a lot!

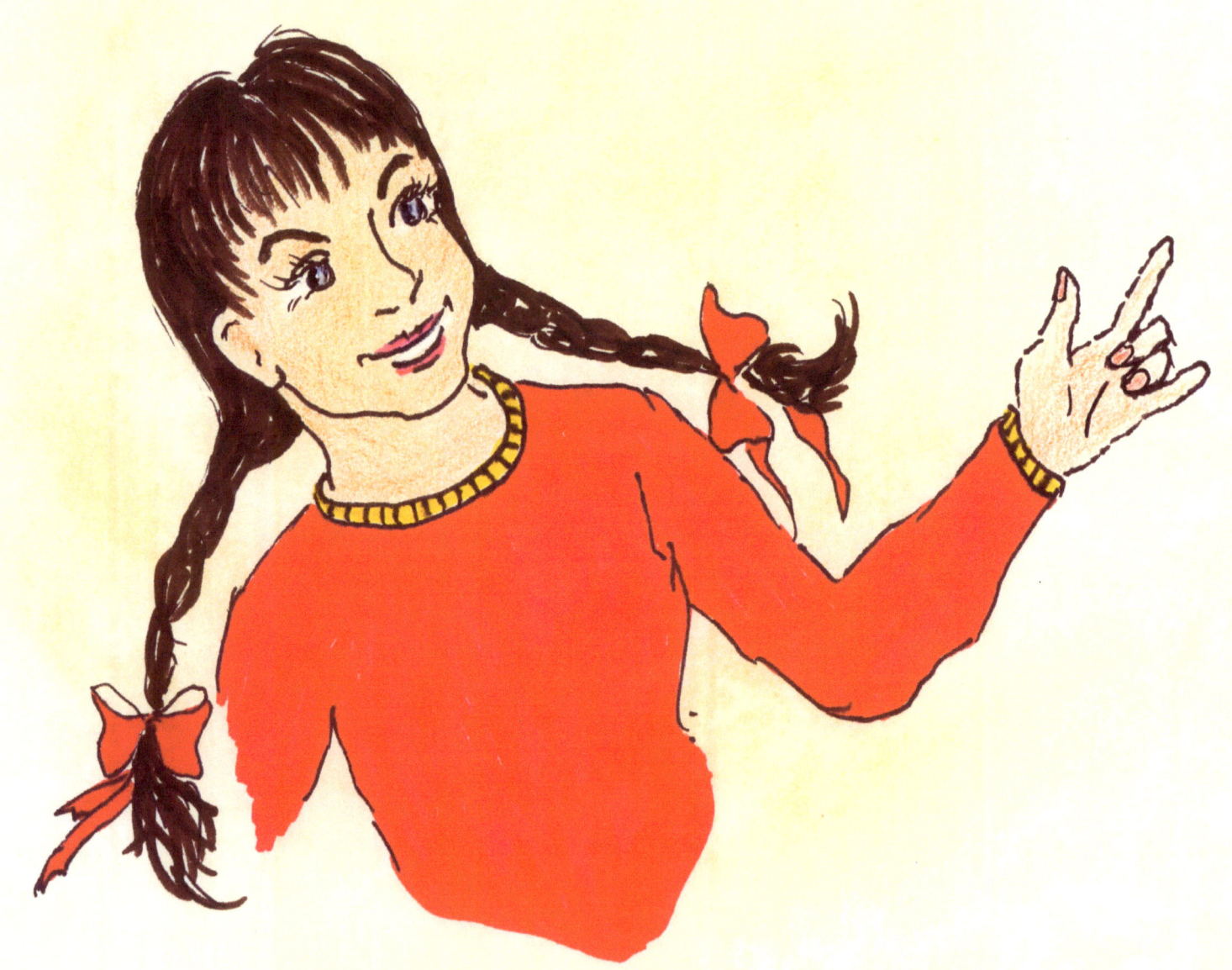

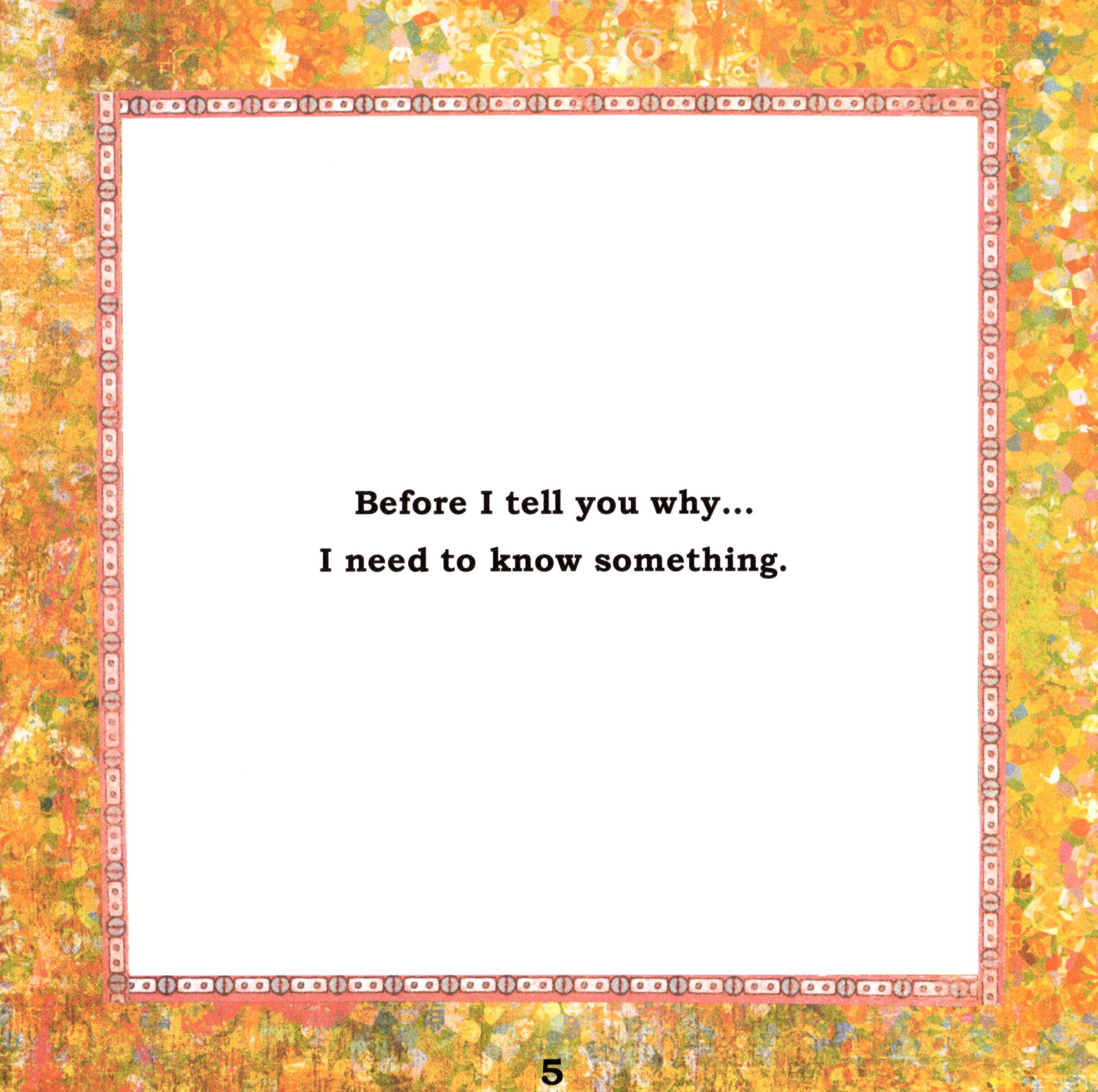

Before I tell you why...

I need to know something.

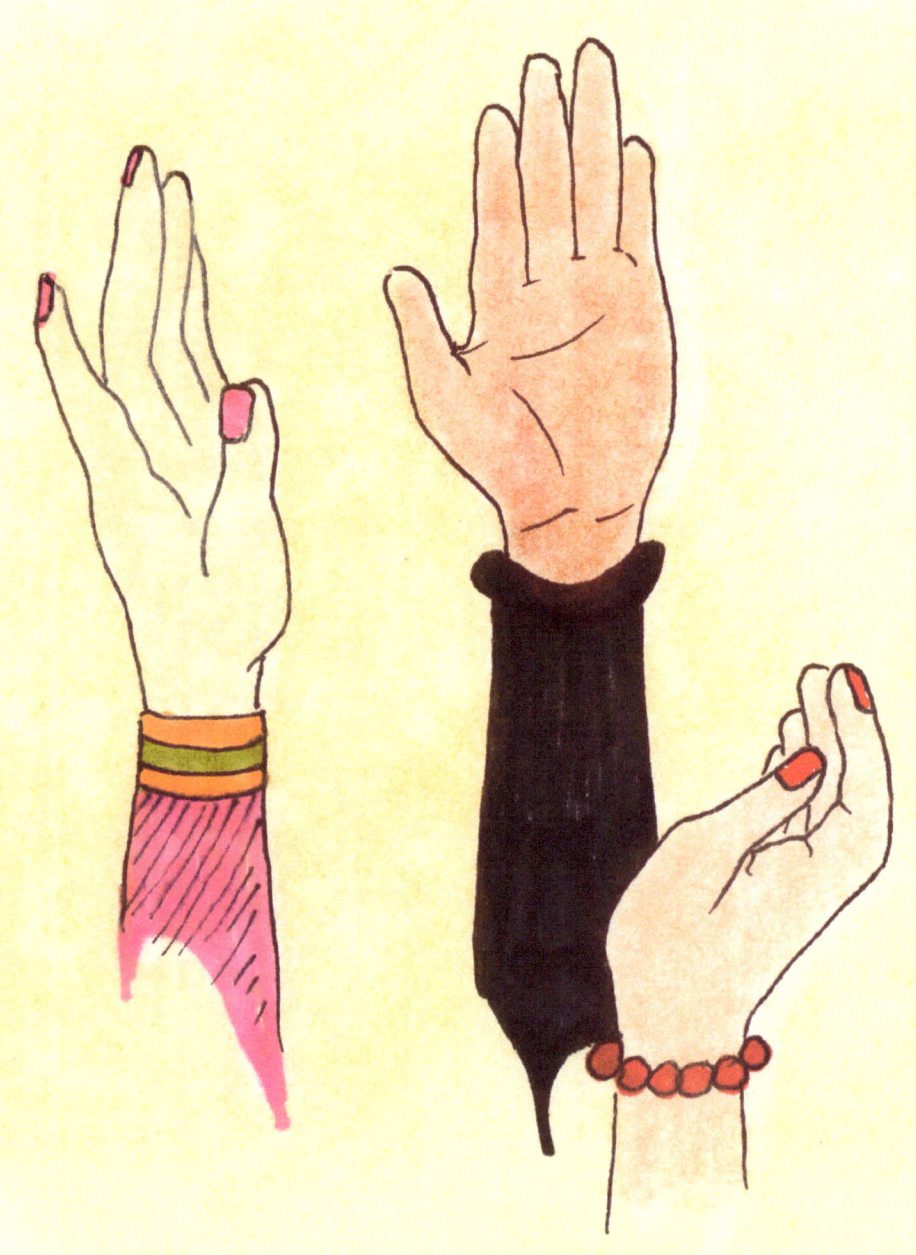

Can you raise your right hand?

then your left hand?

Nice!

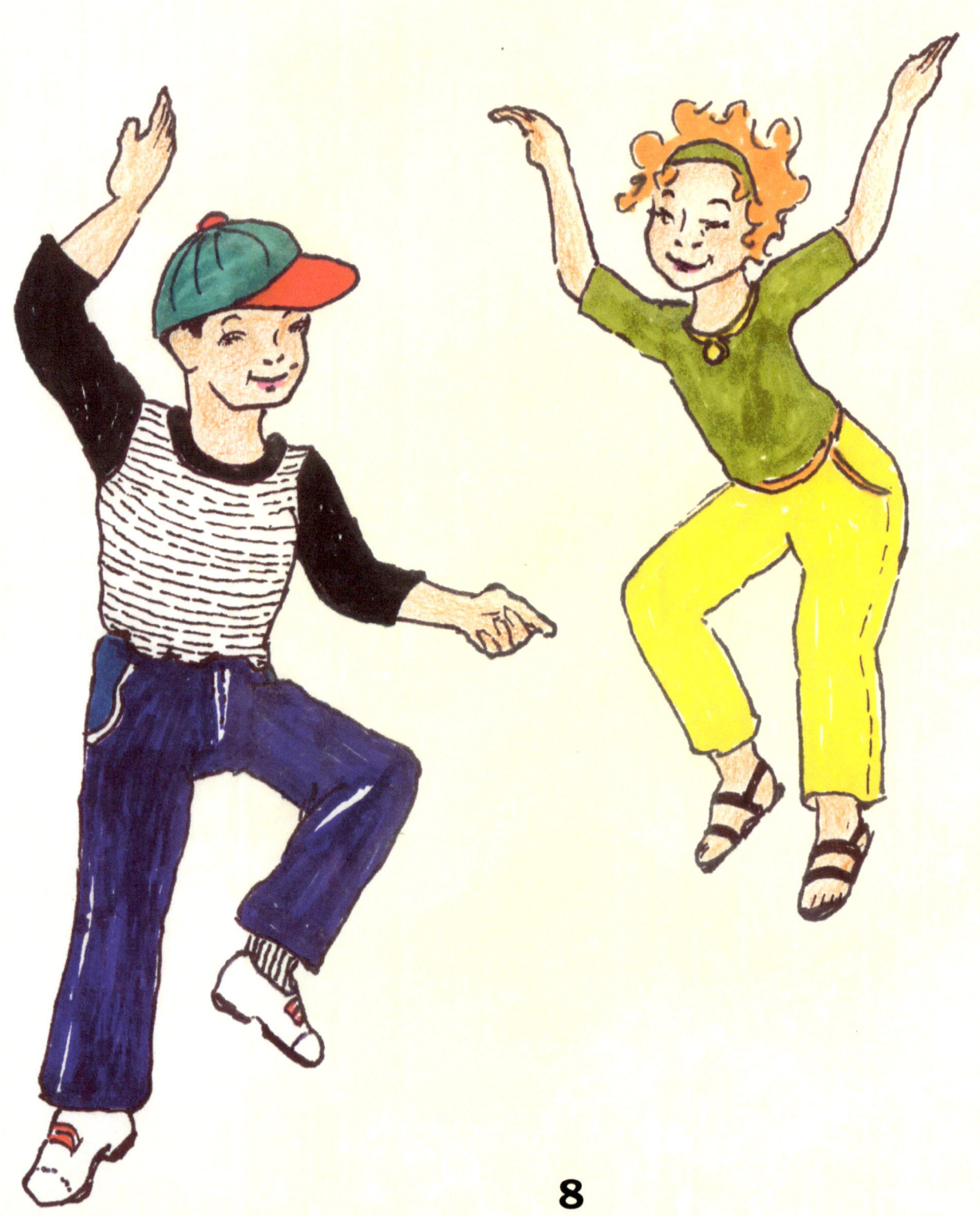

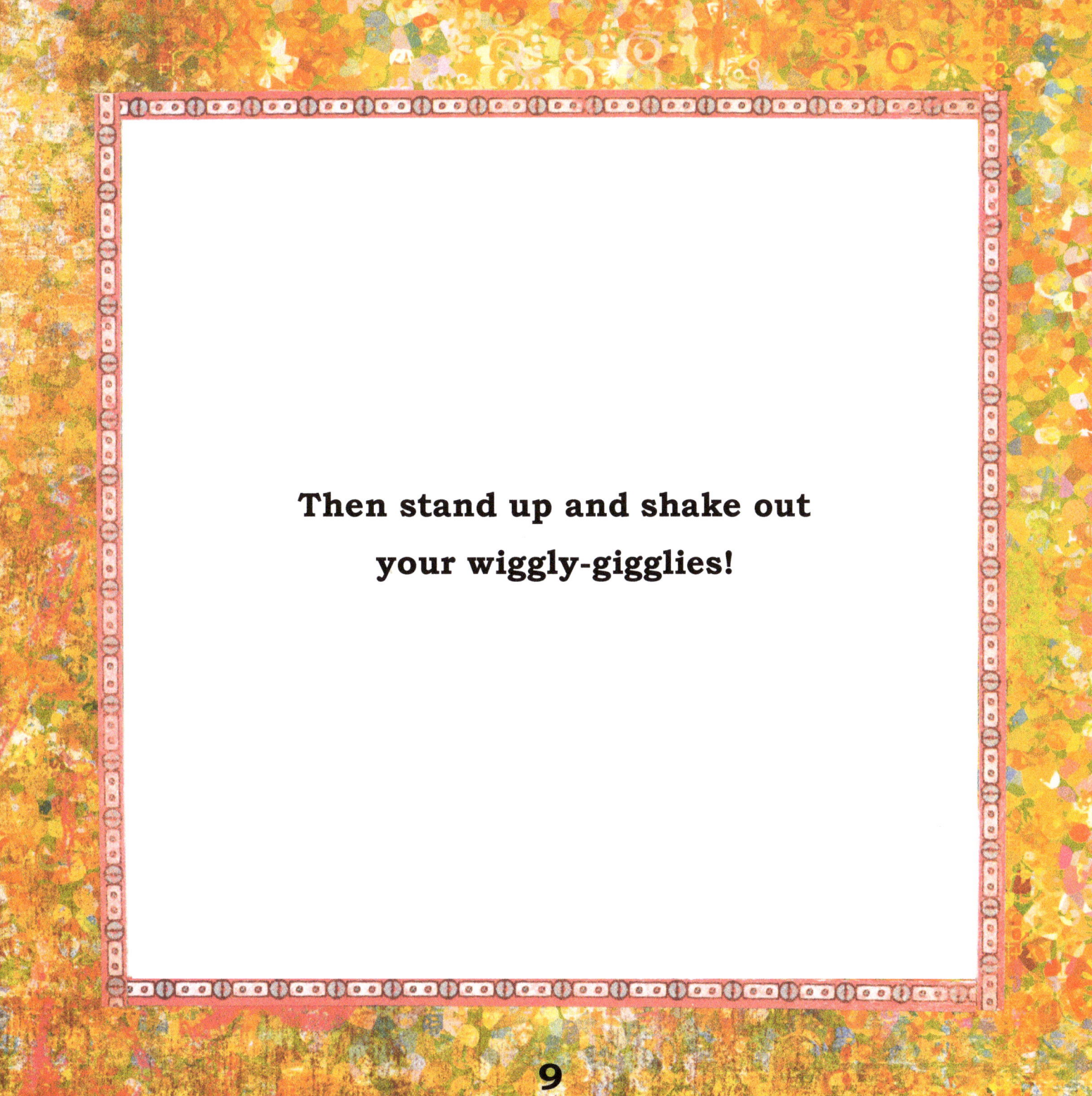

Then stand up and shake out your wiggly-gigglies!

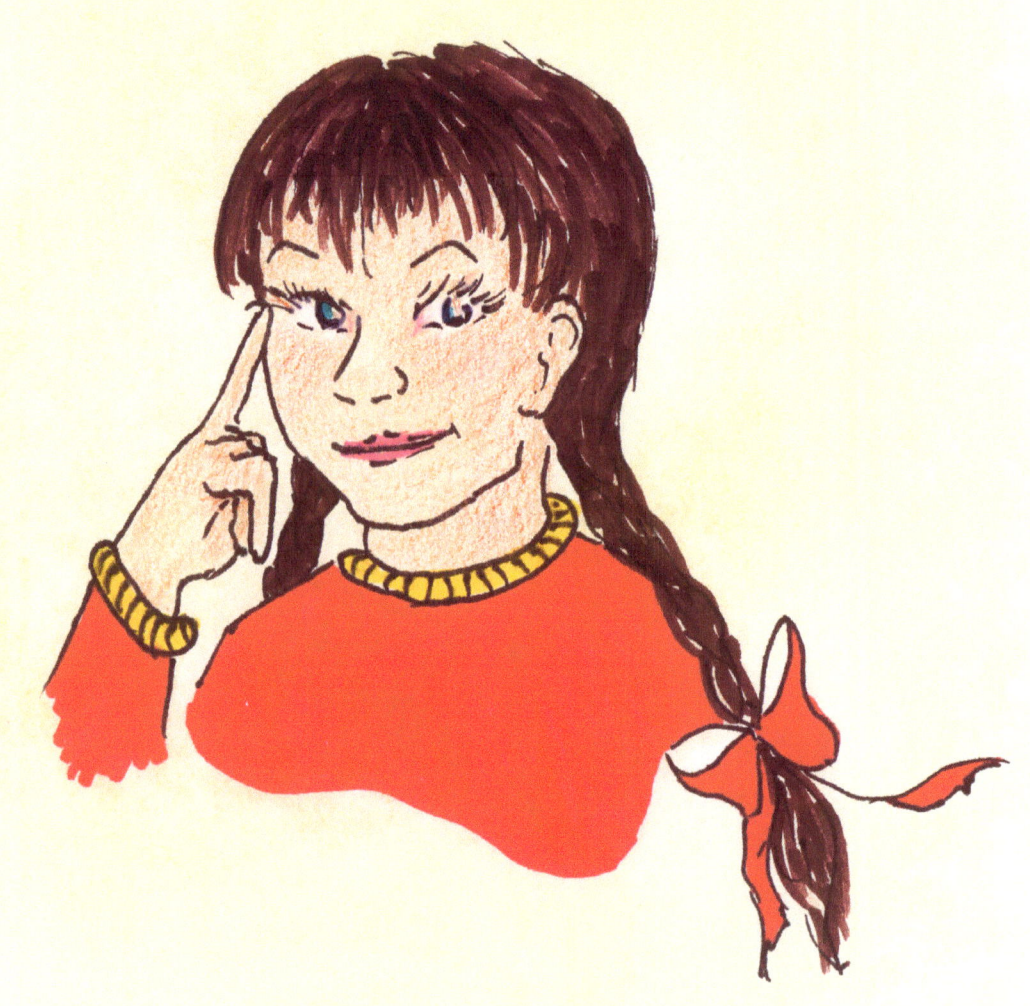

Okay, I think you are

ready for this.

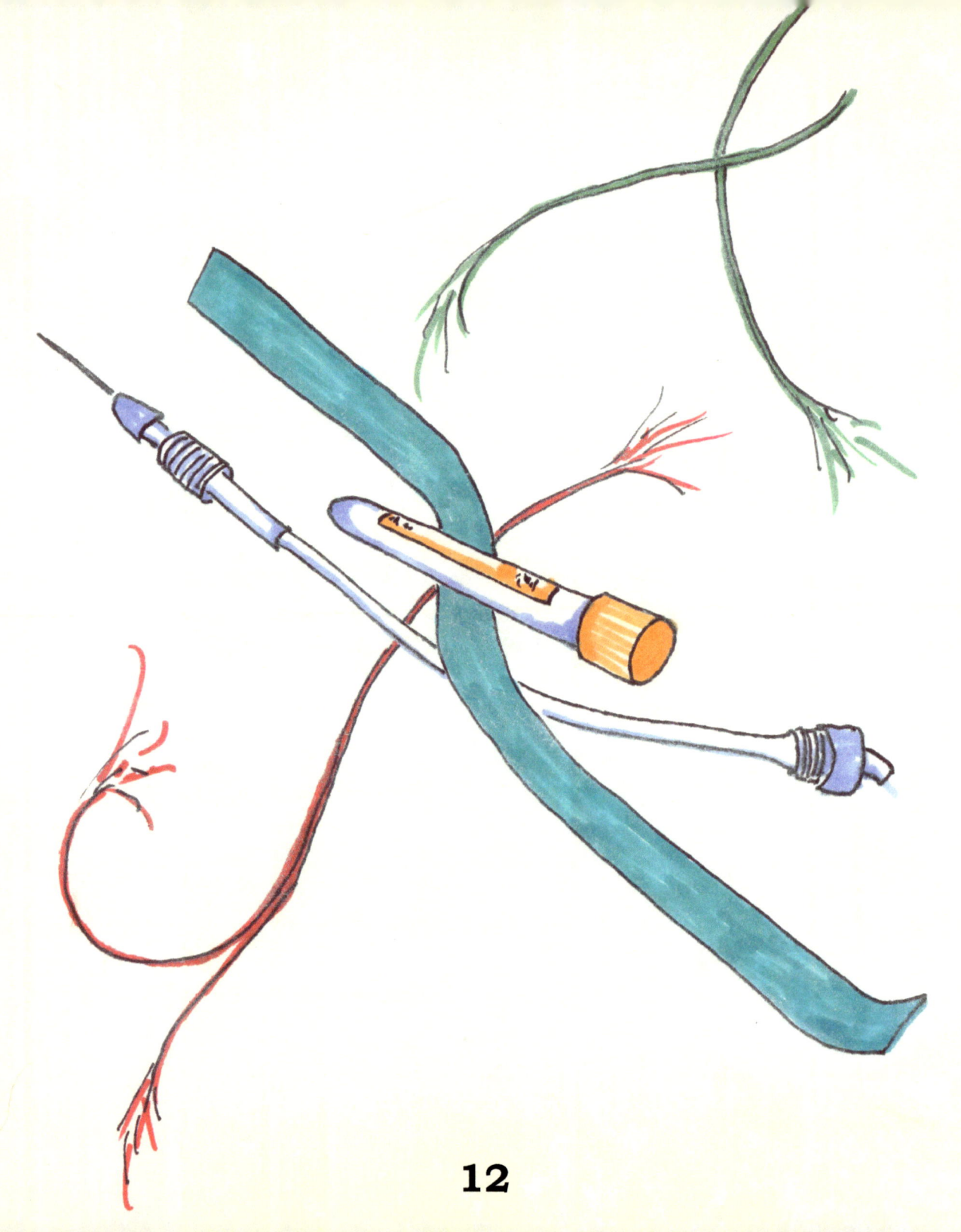

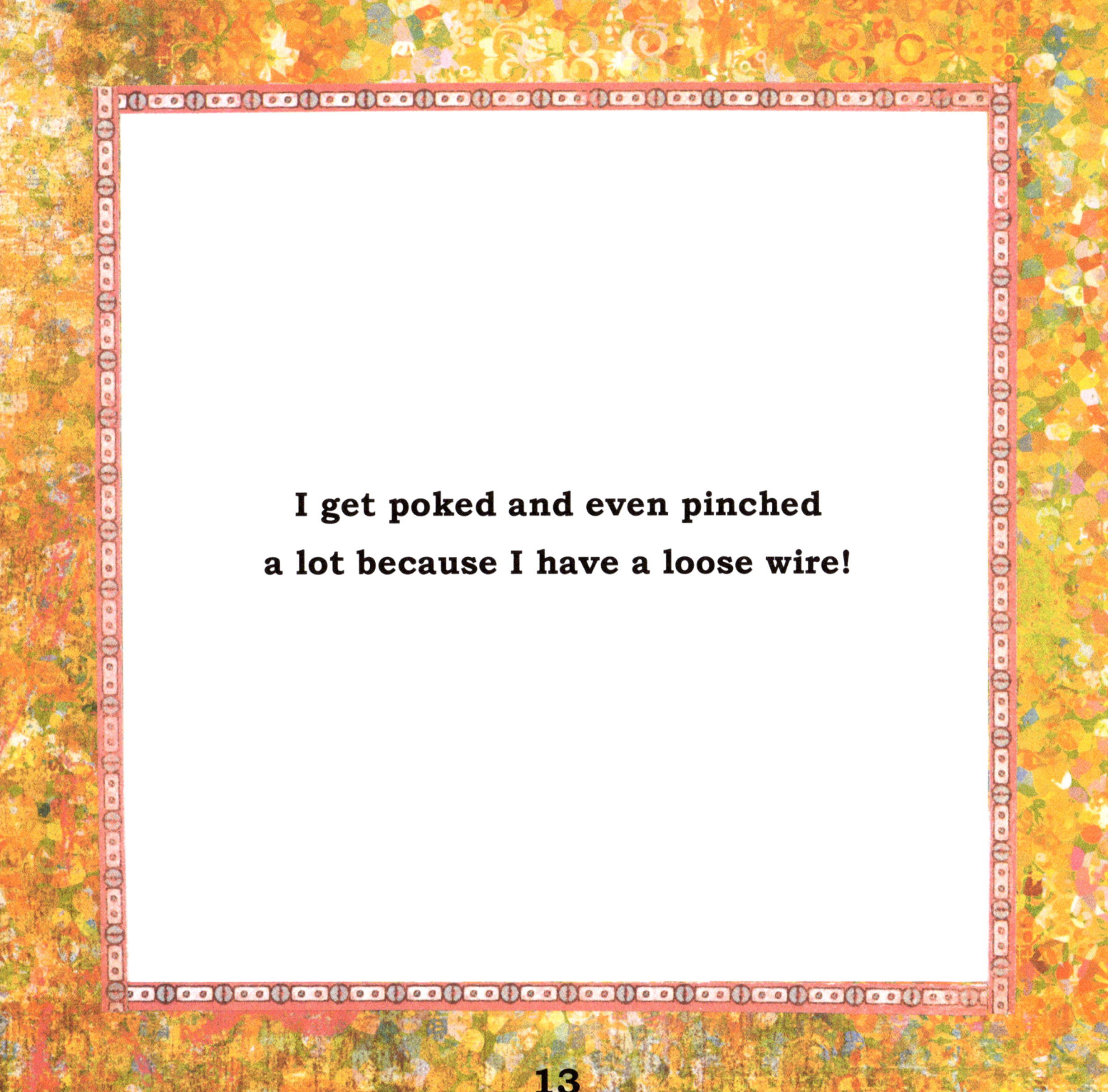

I get poked and even pinched
a lot because I have a loose wire!

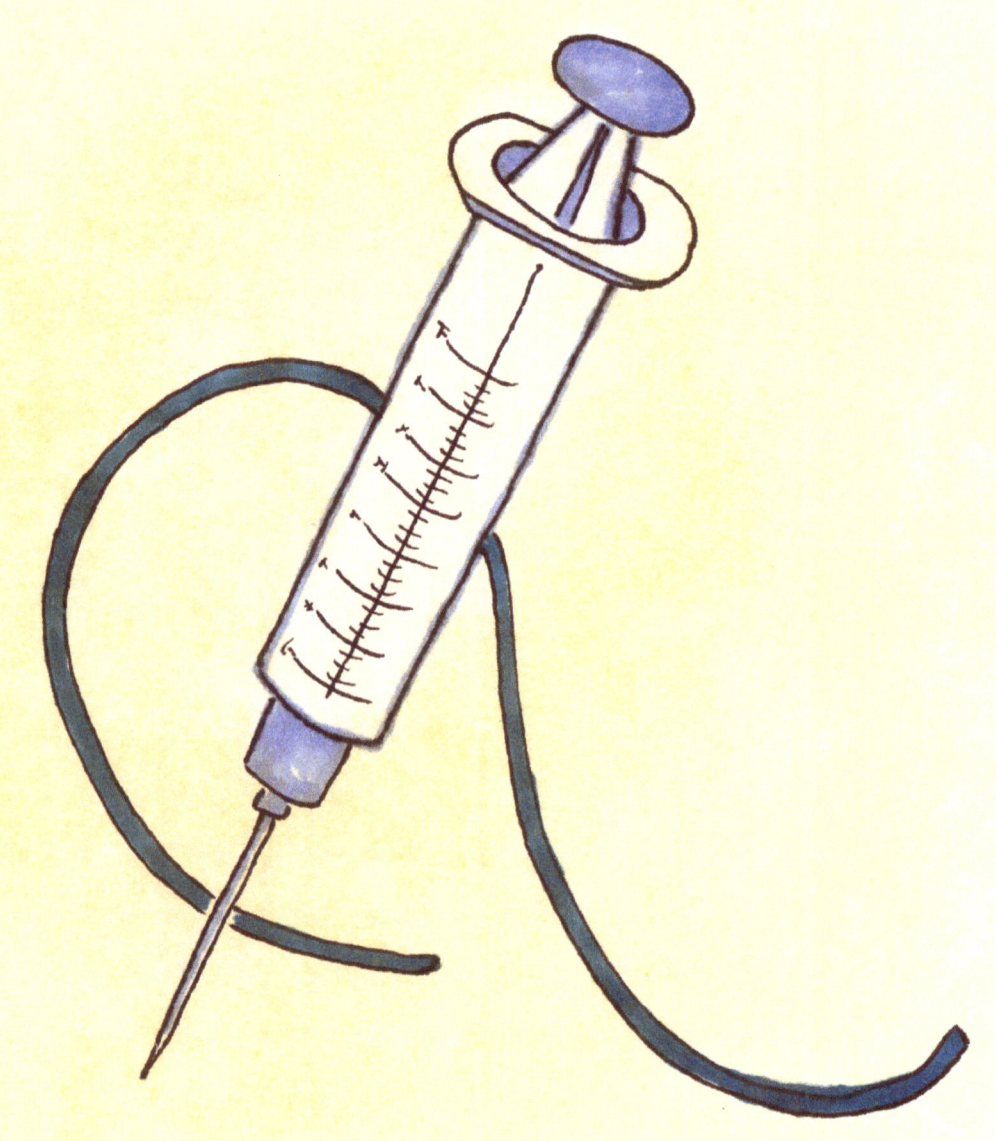

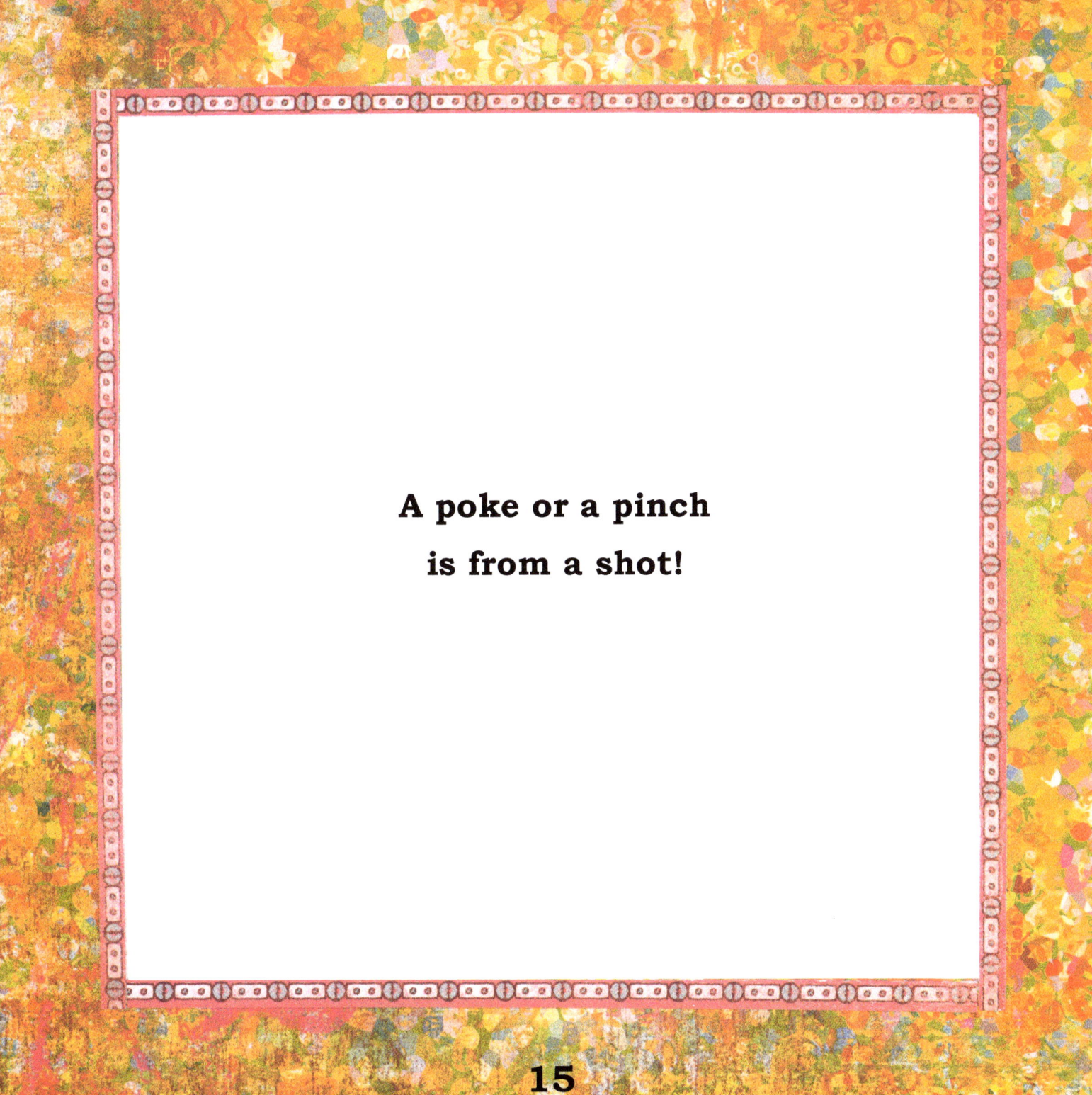

A poke or a pinch
is from a shot!

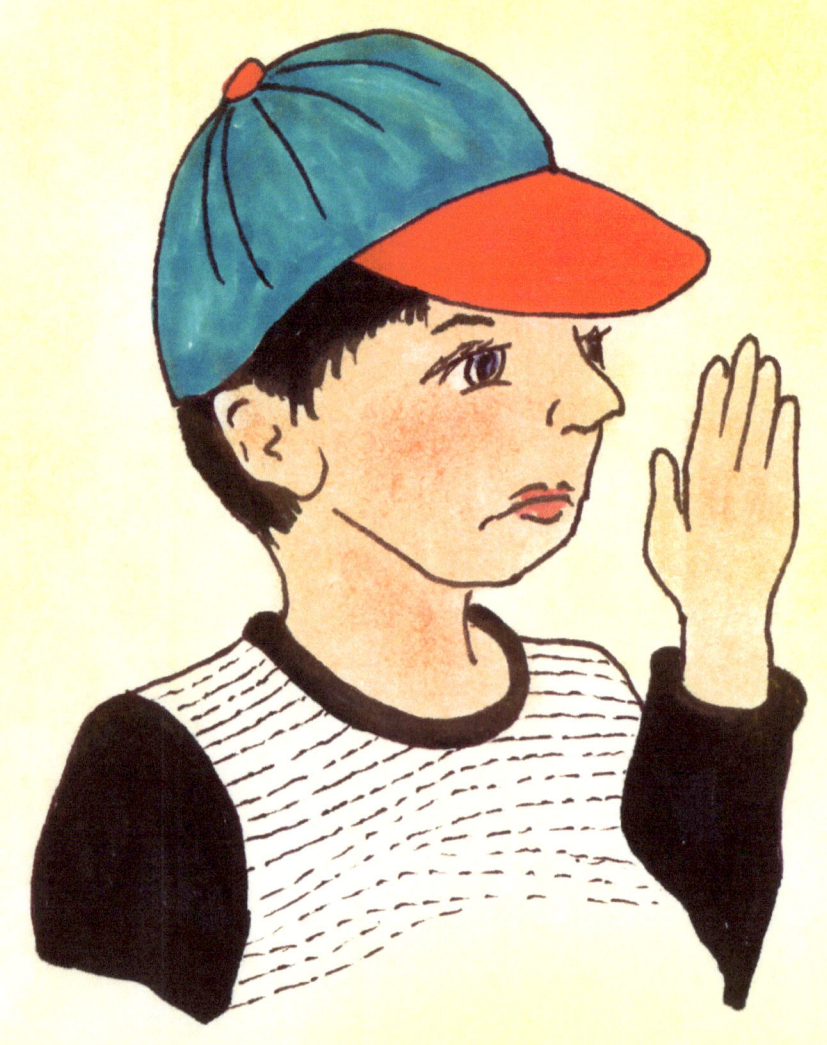

Raise your hand if you've ever had a "poke or a pinch."

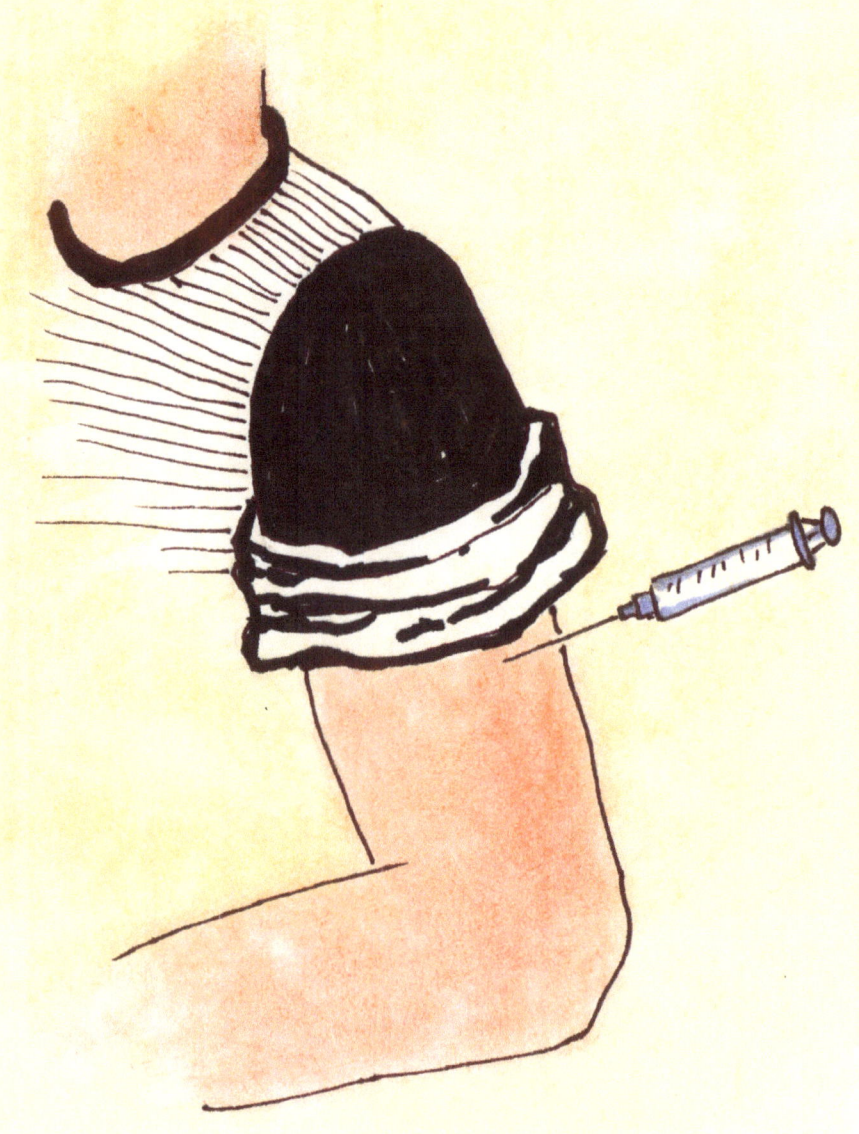

Was your last poke or pinch
on your right arm or left arm?

Still can remember it, right?

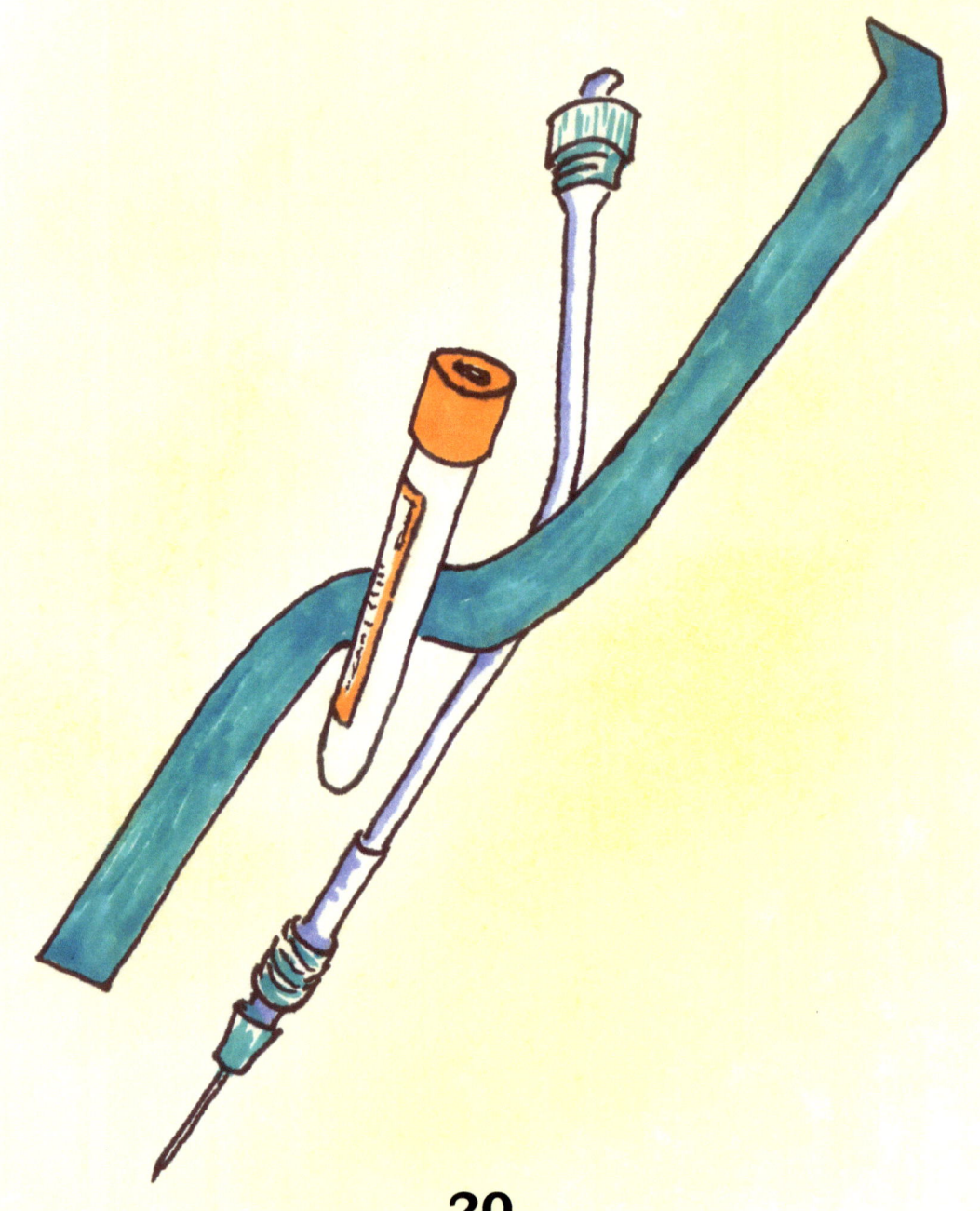

Ever since I was a little kid, I've had to have lots of pokes and pinches.

One day I got another shot and I wondered WHY I had to have so many shots! That's when I learned about my "loose wire."

My bones do not make red blood cells; the needle is the only way to get blood into my body.

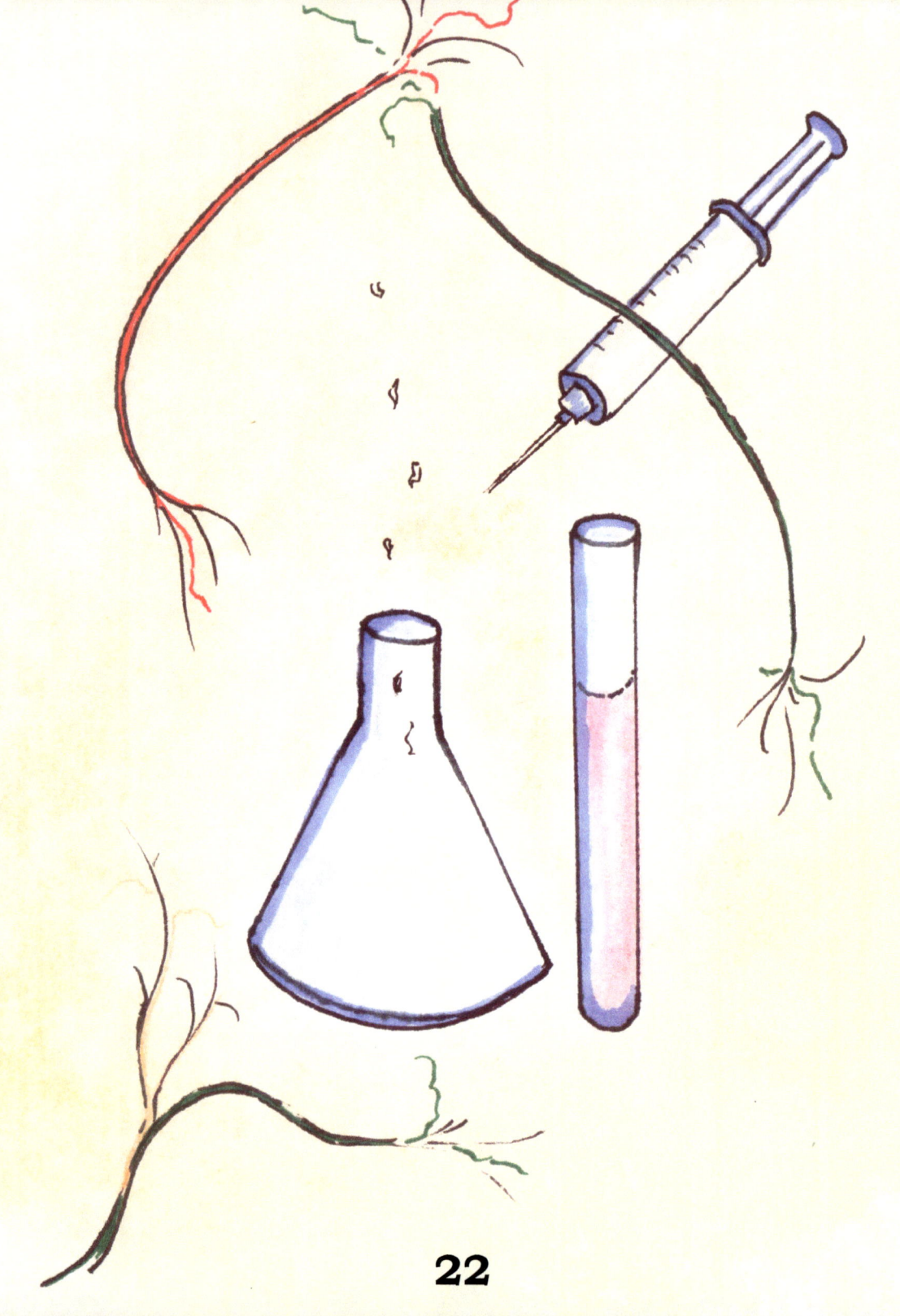

22

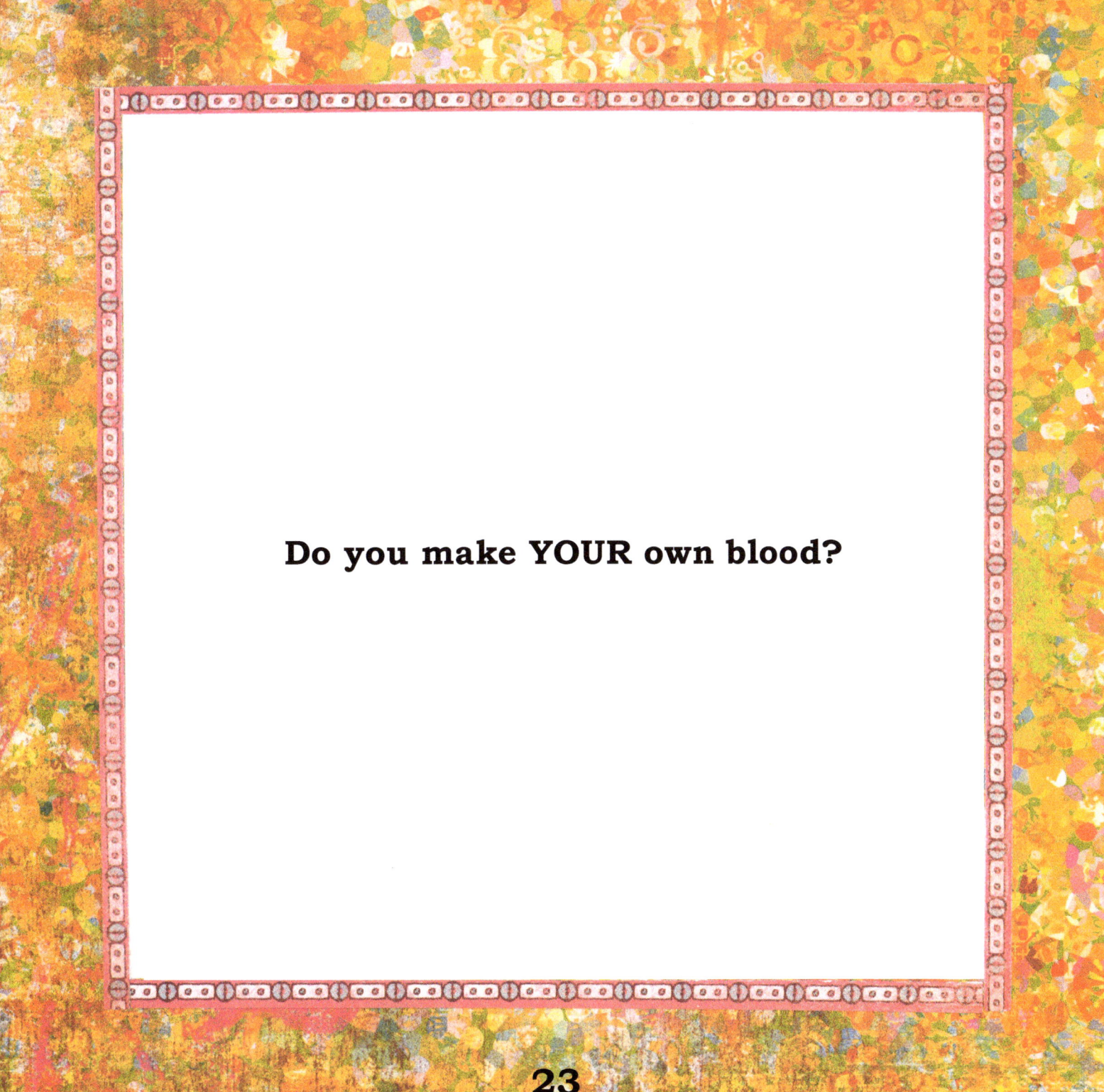

Do you make YOUR own blood?

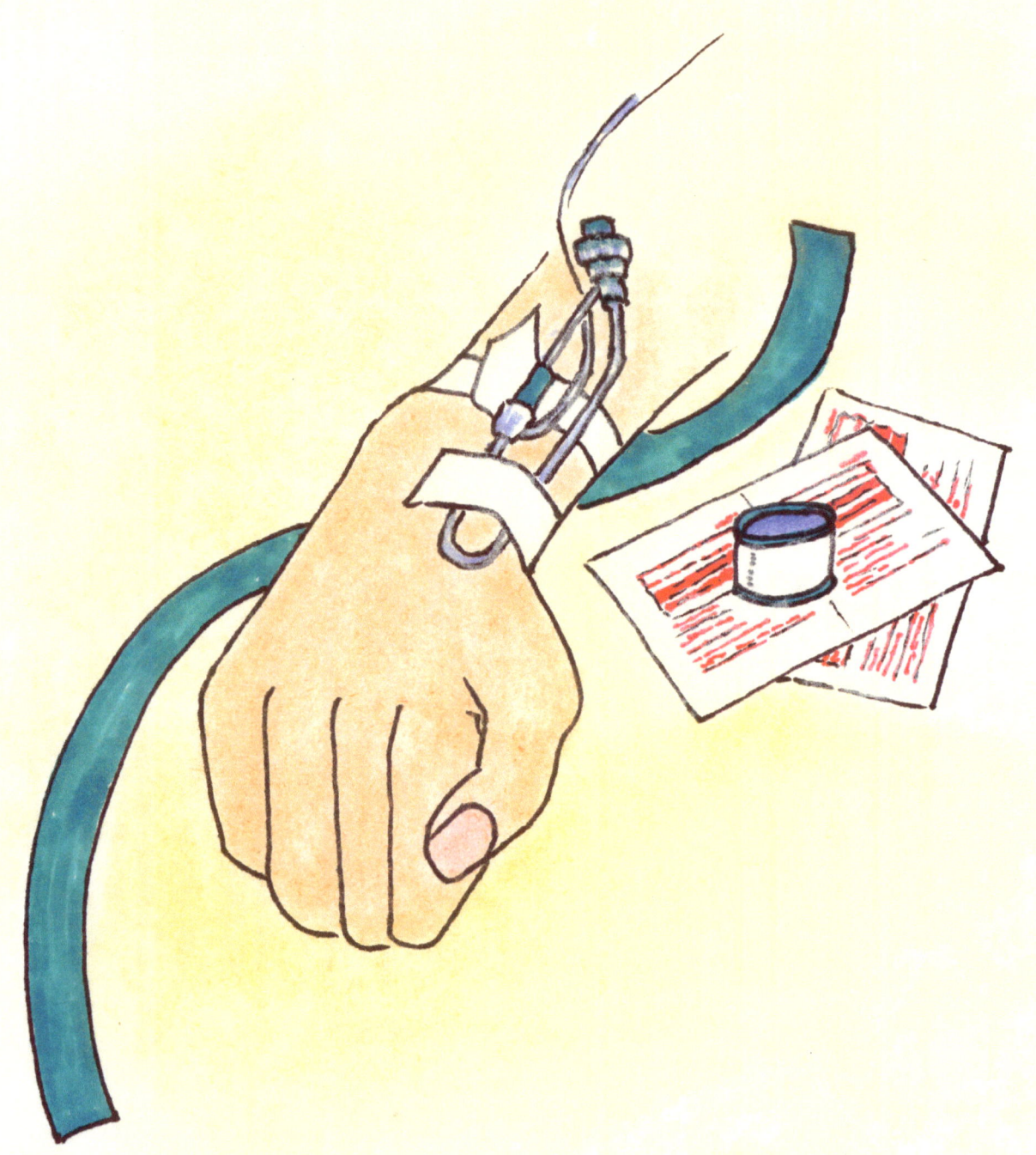

Shots and medicine or things like blood have to go through a needle to get into the body.

Since I do not make my own red blood cells, I have to have lots of "pokes and pinches."

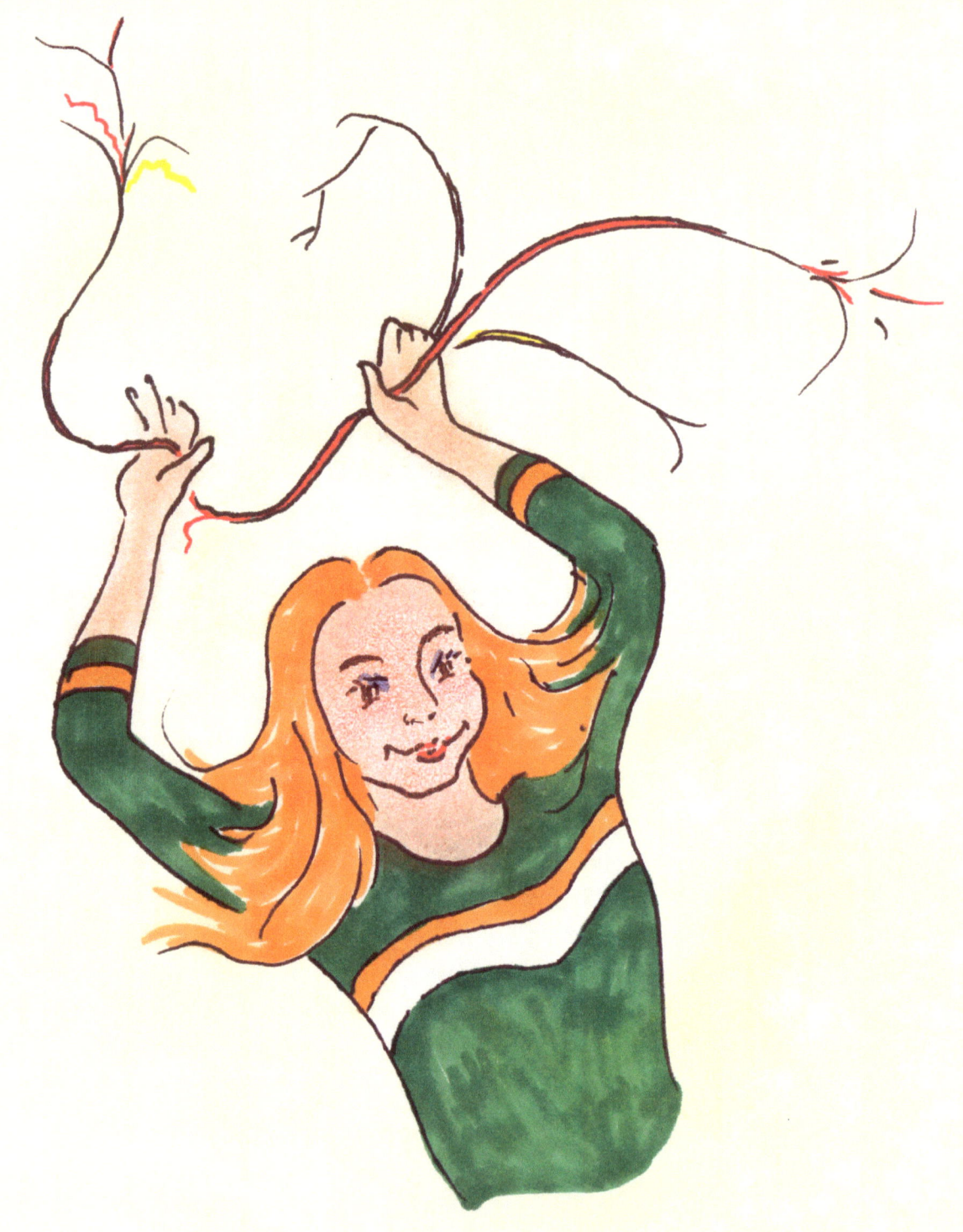

When I was a little kid and asked why my body did not make its own red blood cells, my mom said it was because I had a loose wire; something in my body did not connect.

My body had to have help and my help came from needles, shots, "pokes and pinches." Scary, huh?

Stand up and shake out the Wigglie-gigglies!

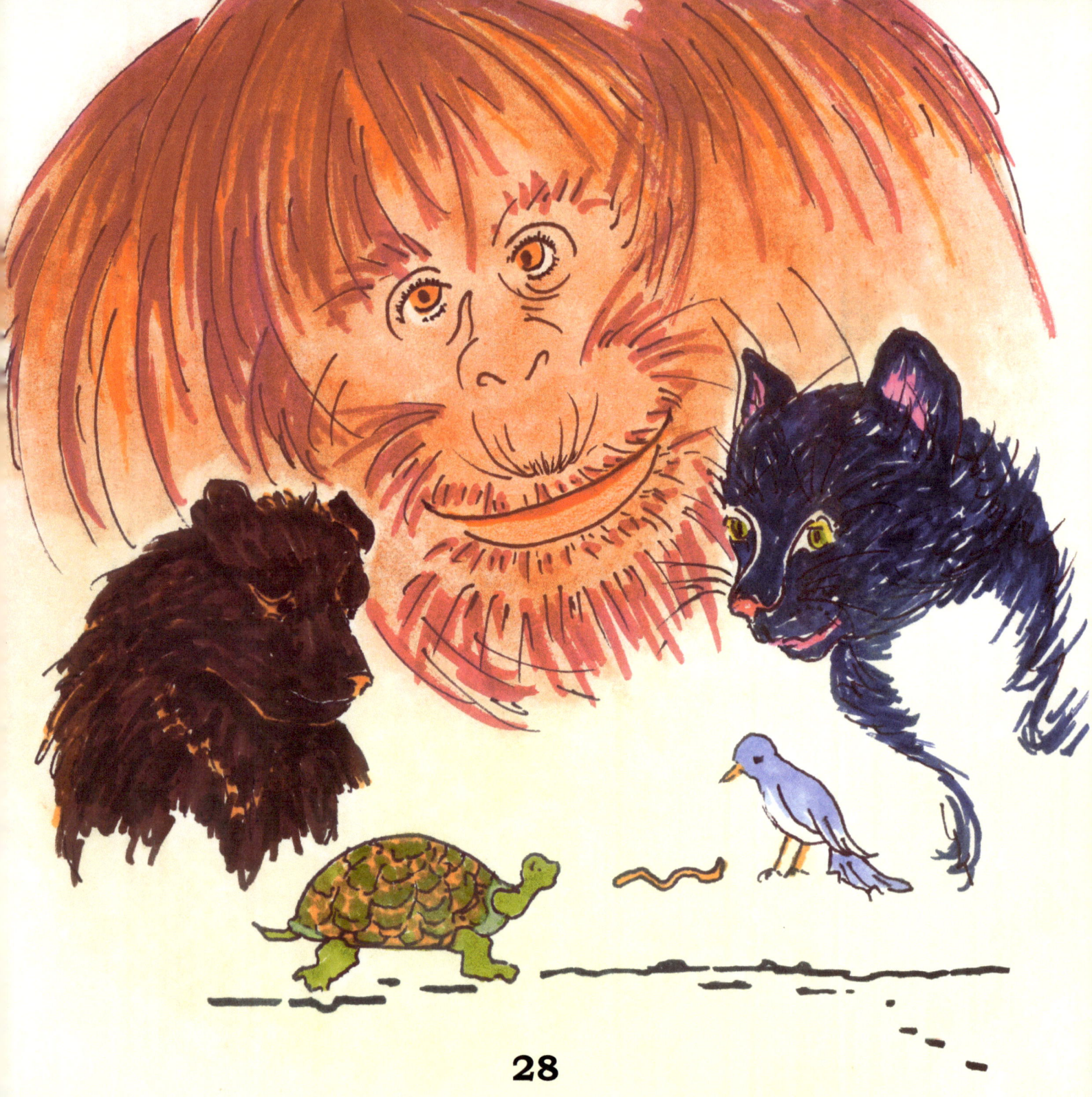

That's when I found out that most living things have to get "poked and pinched." Even animals need shots sometimes!

Needles are one way we get medicine into their bodies too.

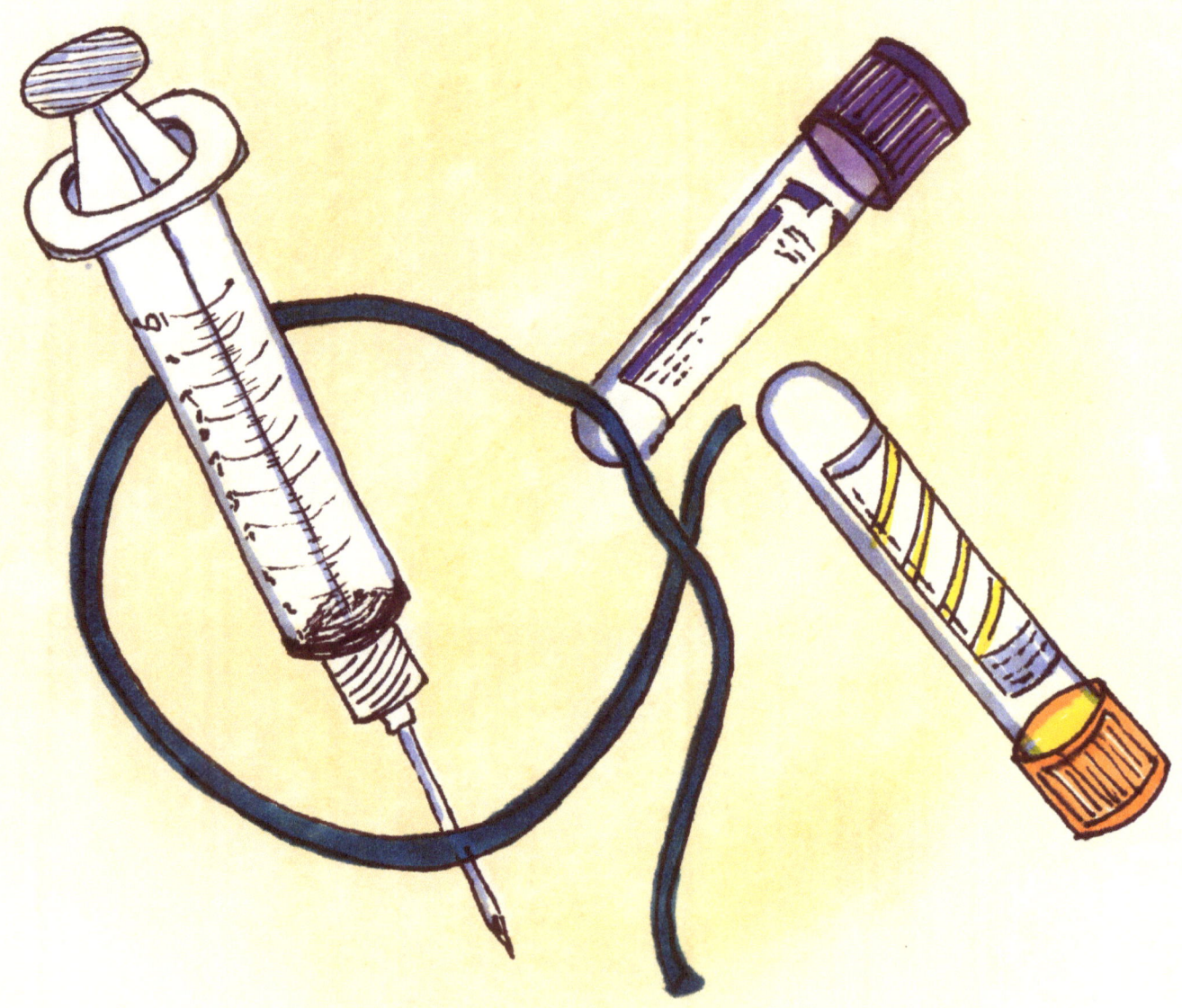

I am not alone, everyone has to be "poked and pinched." You too!

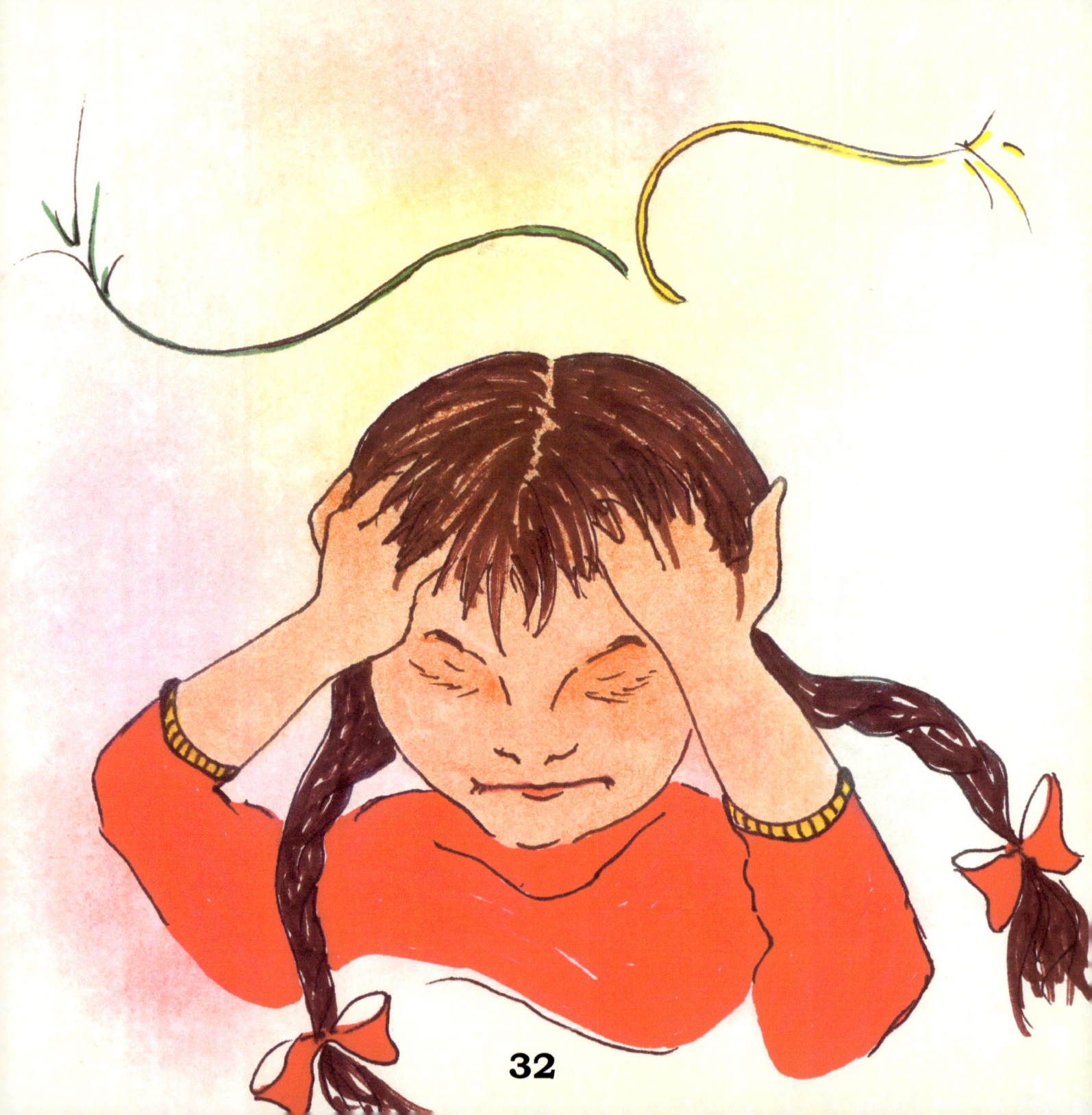

And that's where I learned everyone is born with some kind of "loose wire."

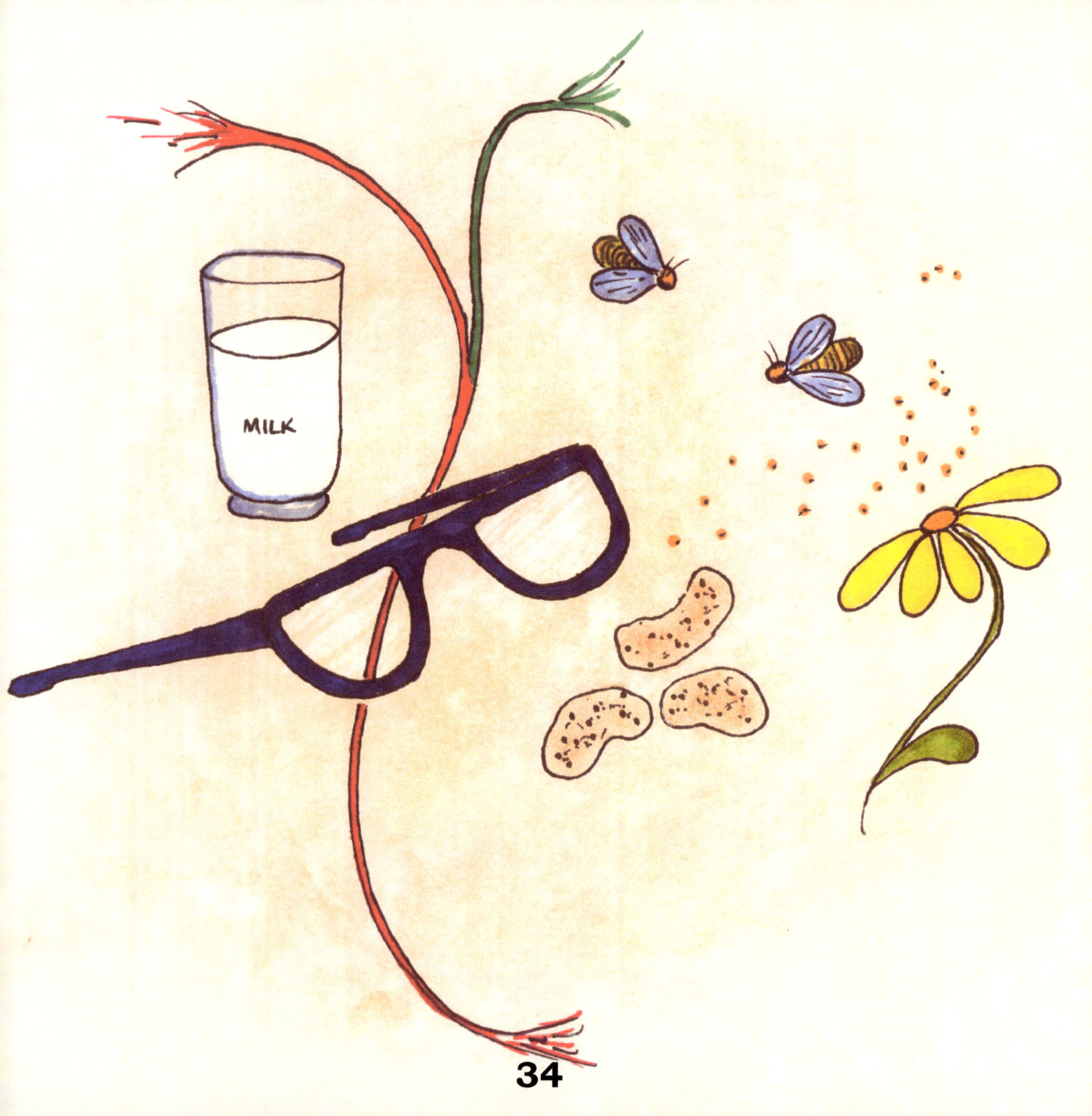

My body does not make red blood cells. Maybe your body has allergies, or you need to wear glasses, or you cannot eat peanuts.

What's YOUR "loose wire"?
Everyone has one!

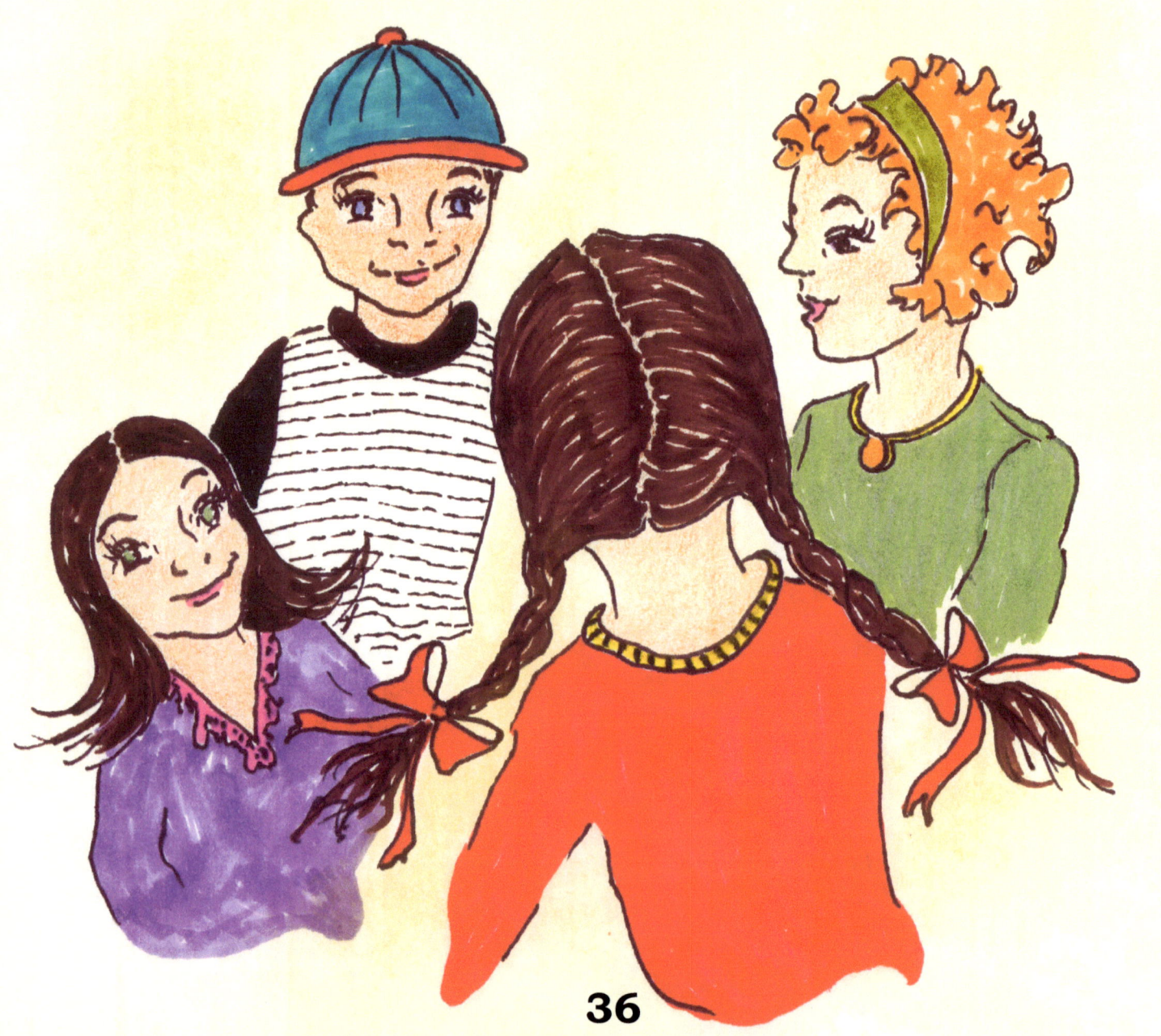

Does your "loose wire" mean you have to have lots of needles too?

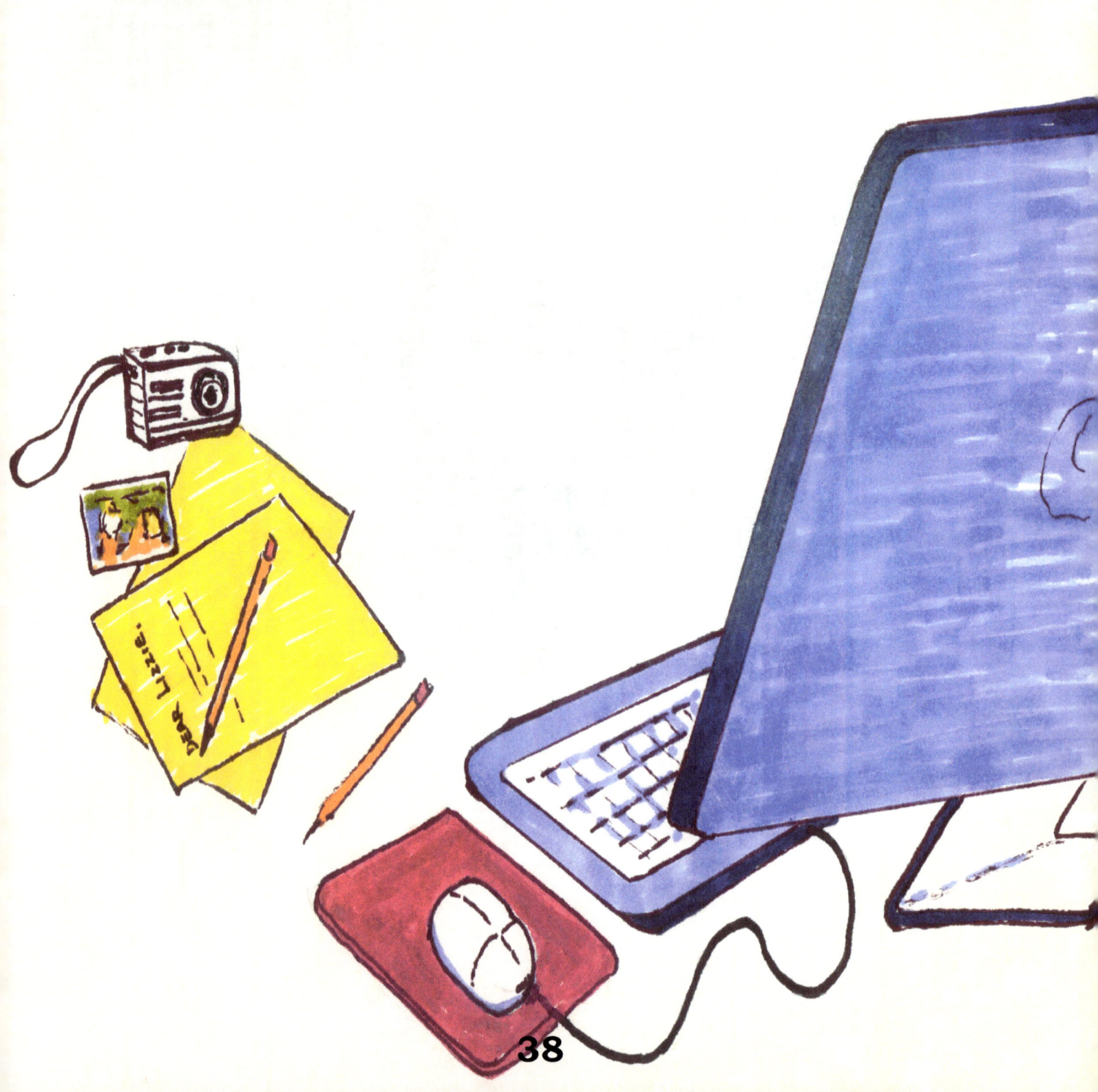

Write to me!

Go to: www.LizzieBell.org

Tell me your "loose wire" story.

Send me a photo of you getting "poked and pinched."

ABOUT THE AUTHOR

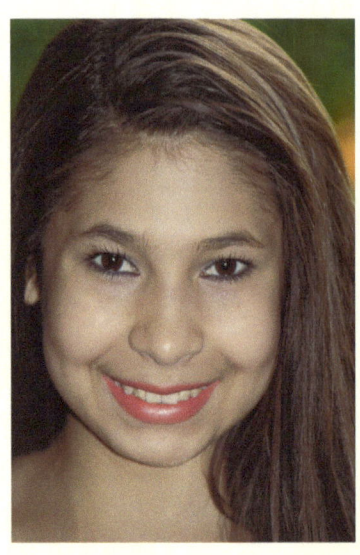

Elizabeth "Lizzie" Bell is a typical girl who loves being with her friends, dancing, traveling and fashion! But she was born with one of the rarest diseases in the world, **Diamond Blackfan Anemia**. Lizzie has been dependent on donated blood and bone marrow most of her life. She is currently awaiting a marrow transplant.

Lizzie tells anyone who will listen about the importance of donating blood and it is working! Between 2009 and 2011, more than 12,000 pints of blood were donated in Lizzie Bell's name and over 1,300 people have joined the National Marrow Registry due to her efforts.

On March 22, 2009, Lizzie's family was featured on **ABC's Extreme Makeover Home Edition**. During the episode, Lizzie did a photo shoot for **Seventeen** magazine and was featured in the May, 2009 issue with fellow American Red Cross celebrity ambassador, Miley Cyrus. To promote World Blood Donor Day in 2010, Lizzie produced a video for kids on Miley's "Get Ur Good On" website. She received the Youth Leadership Award from the Hispanic Women's Corporation later that year.

Following the show, *Team Lizzie Bell* was launched as the Single Voice™ for children whose lives are dependent on blood and marrow donations. Its mission is raising awareness and funds for education, research and advancement in pediatric hematology. Lizzie has published articles in *Latina* magazine, *USA Today*, and *Advance* magazine for medical laboratory professionals. Lizzie is an ambassador for the American Red Cross and was inducted into the Blood Donor Hall of Fame in 2010 at the age of 16. To donate blood, register your marrow, or help to raise funds for *Team Lizzie Bell*, visit Lizzie at **www.LizzieBell.org**.

www.ingramcontent.com/pod-product-compliance
Lightning Source LLC
Chambersburg PA
CBHW042004150426
43194CB00002B/122